Fertility Diet Cookbook for Women

Comprehensive guide for Healthy Recipes for Fertility

Dr. Katrina T. Doles

Copyright © [2023] by [Dr. Katrina T. Doles]

This book is a work of non-fiction. All of the characters, incidents, and dialogue are drawn from the author's personal experiences, interviews, and research. Any resemblance to actual persons, living or dead, or events is entirely coincidental.

While the author has made every effort to provide accurate and up-to-date information, neither the author nor the publisher can be held responsible for any errors or omissions or for any consequences resulting from the use of this information.

Contents

Preface

It had been five years since we exchanged vows and began our joint path of love and devotion. We were content, in love, and flourishing in our jobs, but one unfulfilled dream remained: children. My husband and I experienced the heartbreaking reality of infertility. At the same time, our friends gleefully celebrated the arrival of their children, and our family excitedly anticipated the pitter-patter of tiny feet.

Our infertility experience was defined by several doctor's visits, medical testing, and emotional ups and downs. We looked into several therapy alternatives, seeking answers and solutions that appeared out of reach. But, in the middle of the anguish and uncertainty, we held on to a ray of hope that led us down a route we hadn't explored before: the power of nutrition and the fertility diet.

In our search for solutions, we looked at fertility and diet. We studied books, combed through research papers, and spoke with specialists who underlined the importance of food in reproductive health. This newfound understanding was a surprise, a lifeline we had not anticipated finding. We resolved to take charge of our reproductive journey by adopting a fertility-friendly diet and lifestyle.

The voyage had its challenges. We faced sceptics who questioned the effect of food on fertility, as well as our doubts and fears. But as we progressed along this path, we discovered the incredible power of the right foods to nourish our bodies and souls. We learnt to appreciate the beauty of entire, nutrient-dense foods and the delight of cooking together, each mouthful laced with our shared hope and love.

We started to see improvements as a result of our exploration and perseverance. My menstrual cycle became more regular, my energy levels increased, and I felt rejuvenated. The process was not linear; setbacks happened, but we remained optimistic that we were creating the finest setting for the miracle we desired.

Then, one day, the news we'd been waiting for arrived: an unexpected and priceless positive pregnancy test. Tears of pleasure and surprise came freely, and as we hugged, we realized that our fertility diet had played an essential part in this historic success.

This book, "Fertility Diet Cookbook for Women," concludes our journey filled with hope, love, resilience, and excellent cuisine. We sincerely endeavour to share the information and recipes that brought us to parenting. These pages will serve as a beacon of hope for people struggling with infertility, a source of empowerment through nutrition, and a monument to the human body's extraordinary ability to heal and produce life.

May you discover food for your body and inspiration for your soul as you flip the pages and explore the recipes. Keep in mind that you are not alone on this path. We stand by you, sharing our experience as proof of the power of love, persistence, and the astounding influence of a fertility-friendly diet.

Chapter 1

1.0 Understanding Fertility and Nutrition,

1.1 Fertility and Its Influencing Factors

Fertility, or the capacity to conceive and carry children, is crucial to human existence. It is a journey defined by hope, anticipation, and the desire to generate new life and nurture the next generation. Yet, for many people and couples, the parenting journey is only sometimes smooth and may be plagued with problems and concerns.

Understanding fertility and the variables that control it is a critical first step in navigating the complicated landscape of reproductive health. In this chapter, we go on a voyage of discovery, studying the subtleties of fertility, its relevance in our lives, and the different circumstances that play critical roles in deciding our capacity to conceive.

The Significance of Fertility

Fertility is an emotional, social, and sometimes very personal event, not just a medical procedure. The urge to have children is a universal human desire that transcends cultural, religious, and geographical barriers. It is a desire many people and couples share and promises love, progress, and continuity.

The power to bring a new life into the world demonstrates the human body's resilience and awe. It shows the complicated interaction of hormones, organs, and systems that must all work together for conception. However, fertility is delicate and susceptible to various internal and environmental circumstances.

Factors Affecting Fertility

Fertility is a complicated notion that is impacted by a variety of circumstances. While we may influence some of these elements, others are beyond our control. This chapter delves into the variables that might affect fertility, such as:

Age: The age at which a person or couple tries to conceive may substantially impact fertility. We investigate the biological changes that occur with ageing and their consequences.

Our entire health and lifestyle choices have a significant impact on fertility. We talk about how diet, exercise, and stress affect reproductive health.

Medical issues: Certain medical problems might influence fertility directly or need medical intervention. We look at conditions like polycystic ovary syndrome (PCOS) and endometriosis.

Hormonal Balance: Hormones are the messengers responsible for regulating the menstrual cycle and ovulation. We investigate the delicate hormonal balance in the setting of fertility.

Environmental Toxins and Pollutants: Environmental toxins and pollutants may disrupt fertility. We investigate how these variables may affect reproductive health.

Emotional and psychological factors: Individuals' and couples' emotional and psychological states may impact fertility. Among the things we consider are stress, anxiety, and depression.

Genetics: Our genetic makeup may also influence fertility by affecting aspects like reproductive potential and the risk of hereditary disorders.

1.2 The Nutritional Role in Fertility

Nutrition, often lauded as the foundation of good health, is vital to fertility. It's not just about keeping a healthy weight or having enough food; what you eat may greatly influence your potential to conceive and have a successful pregnancy. This chapter delves into the complex link between diet and fertility, emphasizing how your foods might affect your reproductive health.

Fertility: A Tender Balance

In essence, fertility involves a delicate balance of hormones, body functions, and physiological processes. Several essential factors must exactly coincide for conception to occur. These include the release of a mature egg, healthy sperm, and optimal uterine circumstances for implantation. Each of these factors is influenced differently by nutrition.

Important Nutrients

Because of their direct or indirect functions in reproductive processes, several nutrients are especially crucial for fertility. These nutrients are as follows:

Folate: Folate, also known as vitamin B9, is essential for DNA synthesis and repair. It is necessary during the early stages of pregnancy. Adequate folate consumption lowers the risk of neural tube defects in developing fetuses.
Iron is required for the transfer of oxygen throughout the body. Iron deficiency may cause anaemia, impairing fertility and raising the risk of premature delivery.

Omega-3 Fatty Acids: These beneficial fats help to regulate hormones, reduce inflammation, and improve egg quality. Fatty fish like salmon, flaxseeds, and walnuts are good sources.
Antioxidants, such as vitamins C and E, selenium, and beta-carotene, can protect reproductive cells from free

radical damage. They may boost sperm quality and egg health.

Calcium and Vitamin D: Adequate calcium and vitamin D consumption is necessary for bone health and general wellness. Hormonal balance is also linked to vitamin D. Zinc is necessary for DNA synthesis, immune function, and hormone regulation. It is critical for the reproductive health of both men and women.

Hormone and Nutritional Balance

Fertility is dependent on hormonal balance. Nutrients can influence hormonal regulation, assisting in creating an environment favourable to conception. Maintaining stable blood sugar levels, for example, through a balanced diet, can help to prevent insulin spikes, which can disrupt hormone production. Additionally, certain foods can stimulate the release of hormones that regulate the menstrual cycle and ovulation.

The Weight-Fertility Connection

Weight has a substantial impact on fertility. Fertility problems may occur in underweight and overweight people—nutrition affects not just your weight but also the hormonal signals that govern your appetite and metabolism. A healthy weight achieved by a well-balanced diet may improve fertility.

Fertility-Friendly Eating Strategies

This chapter will examine tactics for following a fertility-friendly diet, such as meal planning, food selection, and portion management. We'll explore how to include fertility-boosting foods in your everyday meals and snacks. Additionally, we'll examine how to overcome food constraints and traverse different nutritional methods in the context of fertility.

As we go further into fertility and nutrition, remember that every person's path is unique. What works for one may not work for another. Nevertheless, by knowing the profound significance of diet in fertility, you may make educated decisions and begin your journey to parenting with confidence and excitement.

1.3 Common Fertility Issues

The road to motherhood is not always easy, and many people and couples have fertility issues. These difficulties may be emotionally and physically draining, yet.
Understanding them is critical in finding answers and realizing your child-bearing ambition. In this chapter, we'll look at some of individuals' most frequent reproductive issues.

1. Inconsistent Menstrual Cycles

Irregular menstrual periods might indicate hormonal imbalances or illnesses like polycystic ovarian syndrome (PCOS). Irregular cycles may make predicting ovulation and the fertile window challenging.

2. Anovulation

Anovulation is the lack of ovulation, which occurs when the ovaries do not produce an egg throughout the menstrual cycle. Because fertilization cannot happen without an egg, this may be a severe obstacle to conception.

3. Inadequate Sperm Count and Quality

Male infertility is often blamed on insufficient sperm count or sperm quality. Lifestyle decisions, toxicity exposure, and underlying medical disorders may all contribute to these problems.

4. Tubal Obstruction

Blocked fallopian tubes may prevent the egg from contacting the sperm, making conception difficult. Infections, scar tissue, or structural anomalies may all cause this.

5. Endometriosis

Endometriosis is a disorder in which tissue comparable to the uterine lining develops outside the uterus. It may cause discomfort, inflammation, and adhesions, impairing fertility.

6. Uterine Problems

Uterine abnormalities like fibroids or polyps might obstruct implantation and pregnancy. Structural problems may need medical intervention or surgery.

7. Fertility Decline with Age

Individuals' fertility typically falls as they age. After the age of 35, this drop becomes more apparent in women. As fertility declines, it might not be easy to conceive and bring a baby to term.

8. Undiagnosed Infertility

Despite extensive testing, the reason for infertility remains unknown in some situations. For couples, this may be a complex and bewildering experience.

9. Lifestyle Considerations

Smoking, excessive alcohol use, poor nutrition, and high-stress levels may all negatively influence fertility in both men and women.

10. Medical Problems

Diabetes and thyroid diseases, for example, might impact fertility by disturbing hormonal balance or triggering other issues.

Obesity and being underweight

Obesity and underweight may also contribute to reproductive issues. Obesity may cause hormonal abnormalities, but being underweight might cause irregular or missing periods.

Prior Reproductive Procedures

Certain medical operations, such as those involving reproductive organs or the removal of one or both fallopian tubes, may influence fertility.

Understanding these frequent reproductive issues is the first step toward overcoming them. It's crucial to remember that therapies, lifestyle modifications, and reproductive interventions are often available to assist individuals and couples in overcoming these challenges. Seeking advice from reproductive health specialists is critical in navigating these issues and building a strategy to reach your fertility objectives.

1.4 How Can This Cookbook Assist You?

Starting a path to maximize fertility via diet is critical in realizing your ambition of becoming a parent. This cookbook is more than just a collection of dishes; it's a complete handbook intended to help you enhance your reproductive health and fertility. This cookbook may assist you on your reproductive journey in the following ways:

1. Recipes for Fertility

This cookbook has a variety of tasty, nutrient-dense meals designed to enhance fertility. Each formula is carefully crafted to include substances that promote hormonal balance, egg and sperm quality, and general reproductive health.

2. Nutritional Details

Understanding the nutritional composition of your meals is critical for optimizing fertility. This cookbook offers thorough dietary information for each dish, allowing you to make educated decisions about the foods you consume and how they may affect your fertility.

3. Meal Preparation

We realize how complex meal planning can be, particularly when attempting to eat for conception. To make your nutritional choices more accessible, we've provided meal planning and recipes. These programs have been carefully crafted to offer balanced, fertility-friendly breakfast, lunch, supper, and snack alternatives.

4. Dietary Advice

This cookbook provides professional advice and practical recommendations to help you manage your nutritional requirements, whether you're following a specific dietary strategy, have dietary restrictions, or want assistance with including fertility-boosting items in your diet.

5. Lifestyle Inclusion

Fertility is affected not just by what you consume but also by how you live. This cookbook discusses lifestyle aspects that might affect fertility, such as stress management, exercise, and sleep. There are suggestions for integrating these variables into your everyday routine to improve your reproductive health.

6. Fertility Education

Knowledge is power, and this cookbook is a recipe book and an instructional resource. Throughout the pages, you'll learn about fertility science, the importance of various nutrients, and the relationship between lifestyle choices and reproductive health.

7. Encouragement and Motivation

Starting a reproductive journey may be emotionally draining. We share inspiring experiences from individuals and couples who have successfully enhanced their fertility via diet and lifestyle changes. These tales may help you keep on track by providing hope, inspiration, and a feeling of camaraderie.

8. Individualization

There are no two fertility journeys similar. This cookbook allows you to tailor your meals and nutritional choices depending on your requirements and tastes. You'll discover alternatives that fit your lifestyle, whether vegetarian, vegan or have specific dietary limitations.

9. Recipes for Every Occasion

Our handbook has dishes for every occasion, from weeknight meals to special events and festivities. You'll discover recipes that cater to your reproductive objectives, whether making a quick and wholesome breakfast or hosting a celebration with friends and family.

10. Laying a Solid Foundation

Finally, this cookbook is about more than simply fertility; it is about laying the groundwork for a healthy lifestyle. The nutrition and well-being ideas discussed in these pages may boost your general health and energy, laying the groundwork for a healthy and satisfying life, with or without children.

With the correct information, support, and nutrition, you can take charge of your fertility journey and maximize your chances of having a healthy, happy kid. This cookbook will be your friend, guide, and source of inspiration as you begin on this incredible journey toward parenting. We wish you success, good health, and pleasure on your fertility journey.

Chapter 2

2.0 Building a Fertility-Friendly Foundation,

2.1 Preconception Nutrient-Rich Foods

Preparing your body for conception is an essential stage in the reproductive process. Nutrition is critical in establishing the ideal environment for a successful pregnancy. This chapter looks at several necessary nutrient-rich foods for preconception health and lays the groundwork for a healthy pregnancy.

1. Vegetables and leafy greens

Vegetables and leafy greens are nutritious powerhouses high in vitamins, minerals, and antioxidants. They include essential nutrients like folate, vitamin C, and vitamin K, which promote conception and a healthy pregnancy. For fertility-boosting advantages, include spinach, kale, broccoli, and Brussels sprouts in your diet.

2. Bright Berries and Fruits

Berries and fruits are high in vitamins, fibre, and antioxidants and are tasty. They aid in regulating blood sugar levels and reducing inflammation, both essential for fertility. Blueberries, strawberries, and citrus fruits are all good options.

3. Seeds and nuts

Nuts and seeds contain healthy fats, protein, and reproductive minerals like zinc and selenium. Almonds, walnuts, flaxseeds, and chia seeds may be added as snacks, smoothies, salads, and yoghurt toppings.

4. Whole grains

Whole grains provide complex carbs and fibre, which assist in keeping blood sugar levels stable and energy levels constant throughout the day. Choose healthy grains such as quinoa, brown rice, and whole wheat pasta to boost your fertility.

5. High-Quality Protein

Protein is required for cell development and repair, especially reproductive cells. To ensure an appropriate intake of this essential nutrient, include lean protein sources such as chicken, fish, tofu, and lentils in your meals.

6. Dairy or Dairy Substitutes

Calcium and vitamin D, crucial for bone health and hormonal balance, are found in dairy products and dairy substitutes such as fortified almond or soy milk. If you want dairy, go for low-fat or non-fat products or fortified alternatives if you're lactose intolerant or prefer a dairy-free diet.

7. Oily Fish

Fish high in omega-3 fatty acids like salmon, mackerel, and sardines, enhance hormonal balance and boost egg quality. These fish also contain vitamin D, which is linked to increased fertility.

8. Leguminosae

Plant-based protein, fibre, and folate are abundant in legumes such as lentils, chickpeas, and black beans. They aid in blood sugar regulation and general reproductive health.

9. Eggs

Eggs are a fantastic source of protein, but they also include critical nutrients such as choline, which is necessary for prenatal brain development. Include eggs in your diet as part of a well-balanced preconception nutrition strategy.

10. Lean meats

Lean meats, such as lean beef and skinless chicken, are rich in protein and vital minerals such as iron and zinc. These nutrients are essential for fertility as well as general health.

11. Avocado

Avocado is a high-nutrient fruit high in monounsaturated fats, vitamin E, and folate. It helps to regulate hormones and offers critical nutrients for reproductive health.

Incorporating these nutrient-dense foods into your preconception diet may help your body prepare for pregnancy. Remember that a diverse and balanced diet is essential for fertility since it delivers various nutrients. Consult a healthcare practitioner or a qualified dietician for tailored advice and suggestions based on your specific requirements and health state.

2.2 Hormone Balance with the Right Diet

Hormonal balance is essential in fertility because hormones regulate the menstrual cycle, ovulation, and general reproductive health. Your food may have a significant impact on your hormone levels.

Function, which affects your capacity to conceive. This chapter examines how the appropriate food may help you achieve hormonal balance and assist your reproductive journey.

Hormones function in the body as messengers, coordinating numerous processes such as the menstrual cycle and ovulation. Hormone imbalance may cause irregular menstrual periods, anovulation (lack of ovulation), and reproductive issues. The appropriate diet may benefit in the following ways:

1. Controlling Insulin Levels

Blood sugar control is critical for hormonal equilibrium. Insulin fluctuations may result in insulin resistance, which has been related to illnesses such as PCOS. Focus on the following while managing insulin levels:

- **Complex Carbohydrates:** To help balance blood sugar, choose whole grains, lentils, and high-fiber meals.

- **Healthy Fats:** Consume avocados, almonds, and olive oil to help decrease carbohydrate absorption.

- **Protein:** Include lean protein sources to help regulate blood sugar.

2. Promoting Estrogen Balance

Estrogen dominance or abnormalities in the estrogen-to-progesterone ratio may cause menstrual cycle disruption. Consider the following to enhance estrogen balance:

- **Cruciferous Vegetables:** Broccoli, cauliflower, and kale contain estrogen-metabolizing chemicals.

- **Fiber:** A high-fiber diet may help the body eliminate excess estrogen.

- Omega-3 fatty acids have been shown to help decrease inflammation and promote hormone balance.

3. Promotion of Progesterone Production

Adequate progesterone levels are required for a healthy menstrual cycle and optimal pregnancy. Focus on the following to boost progesterone production:

- **Vitamin B6:** Foods high in vitamin B6, such as chicken, bananas, and spinach, may aid in hormone production regulation.

- **Zinc:** Zinc-rich foods such as lean meats, nuts, and seeds may help promote hormone function.

- **Magnesium:** Magnesium-rich meals such as leafy greens and almonds may aid in generating progesterone.

4. Thyroid Health Promotion

The thyroid gland is essential for hormone regulation. Consider the following to help your thyroid health:

Iodine: Seaweed, salmon, and iodized salt contain iodine, which is necessary for thyroid function.
Selenium is found in Brazil nuts, healthy grains, and lean meats and is essential for thyroid function.
Limiting Goitrogens: When ingested excessively, several foods, such as cruciferous vegetables and soy, might interfere with thyroid function. Moderation is essential.

5. Reducing Stress Hormones

Hormonal equilibrium may be disrupted by stress. Dietary stress management entails:

Eating frequent, balanced meals may help normalize blood sugar levels and minimize stress.

Mindful Eating: Practicing mindful eating may help you become more aware of your body's hunger and fullness signals, which can help you reduce stress-related eating.

6. Detoxification and Hydration

Adequate hydration aids the body's natural detoxification processes, eliminating excess hormones and toxins. Drink lots of Water and think about herbal teas and meals like citrus fruits to help your liver cleanse.

7. Herbs and supplements

A healthcare provider may offer vitamins and herbal therapies to promote hormonal balance in specific circumstances. Before using vitamins or herbs, always speak with your doctor.

Remember that establishing a hormonal balance with nutrition may take some time, and individual responses may vary. Monitoring your menstrual cycle and consulting with a healthcare physician or a certified dietitian may assist you in fine-tuning your food strategy to meet your hormonal demands and improve your fertility.

2.3 Weight Management for Optimal Fertility

Maintaining a healthy weight is critical for improving fertility and increasing the likelihood of a successful pregnancy. Because underweight and overweight states may influence reproductive health, weight management is an integral part of your fertility journey. In this chapter, we look at the relationship between weight and fertility and provide tips on achieving and maintaining a healthy weight for optimum fertility.

The Relationship Between Weight and Fertility

Both men's and women's fertility are affected by their weight. Extreme weight gain or loss might alter hormonal balance, menstrual cycles, and general reproductive health.

1. Obesity and Fertility

Being underweight, generally characterized by a low BMI, may result in irregular or missing menstrual periods and anovulation (lack of ovulation). Low body fat levels may impair the body's capacity to create the hormones required for conception. To address this:

Balanced Nutrition: To promote healthy weight growth, focus on a well-rounded diet containing various nutrient-dense foods.

Caloric Intake: Ensure you get enough calories to sustain your basal metabolic rate and reproductive health.

Healthy Fats: To promote hormone production, include healthy fats from sources such as avocados, almonds, and olive oil.

Consult a Healthcare physician: To develop a tailored dietary plan for healthy weight gain, seek advice from a healthcare physician or registered dietitian.

2. Obesity and Fertility

As indicated by a high BMI, being overweight may contribute to insulin resistance, hormonal imbalances, and illnesses such as polycystic ovarian syndrome (PCOS), which can pose reproductive issues. To address this:

Balanced Diet: Eat a diet rich in whole grains, lean meats, fruits, and vegetables while reducing processed foods and added sweets.

Exercise regularly to reduce weight, increase insulin sensitivity, and improve general health.

Portion Control: Watch your portion proportions to prevent consuming too many calories.

Moderate Weight Reduction: Rather than severe diets that might alter hormone balance, aim for average and sustained weight reduction.

Consult a Medical Professional: Consult with a healthcare physician or qualified dietitian to design a weight-management strategy that is safe and effective for you.

3. Male Fertility and Weight

Male fertility is similarly affected by weight. Overweight and obese males may have poor sperm quality and hormonal abnormalities. Maintaining a balanced diet, participating in regular physical exercise, and avoiding excessive alcohol and cigarette use are all male weight control measures.

4. Progress Monitoring

Monitoring your weight and menstrual cycles (for women) regularly will help you gauge your progress. But remember that weight is just one part of overall health and fertility. Other health markers include more energy, regular menstrual periods, and better mental well-being.

5. Seeking Help

Weight loss for fertility is a process that may need the assistance of healthcare doctors, licensed dietitians, and even mental health professionals. Feel free to seek advice and help suited to your needs and circumstances.

6. Patience and perseverance

It may take time and work to achieve and maintain a healthy weight. Be patient with yourself and be dedicated to adopting long-term lifestyle changes that will help you achieve your reproductive objectives. Remember that the ultimate aim is to improve your general health and well-being to increase your chances of conceiving and having a safe pregnancy.

You may favourably affect your fertility and boost the probability of a successful pregnancy by trying to acquire and maintain a healthy weight.

2.4 The Effects of Hydration on Reproductive Health

While we frequently identify optimal hydration with overall health, it's vital to remember that enough water consumption is crucial for reproductive health and conception. This chapter discusses the significance of hydration and how it may benefit your reproductive system and overall fertility.

Hydration's Importance in Reproductive Health

Hydration is necessary for a variety of biological activities, including those directly relevant to reproductive health:

1. Cervical Mucus Quality: Hydration impacts the production and consistency of cervical mucus. Cervical mucus is necessary for fertility because it creates an environment conducive to sperm movement. Your cervical mucus is more likely to be of high quality when you are well-hydrated, assisting sperm on their trip to reach the egg.

2. Hormone management: Hormones are essential in menstrual cycle management and ovulation. Adequate hydration aids the body's capacity to maintain hormonal balance, supporting regular menstrual cycles and appropriate reproductive system function.

3. Blood Flow: Hydration aids in the maintenance of average blood circulation, which ensures that the reproductive organs get an appropriate quantity of oxygen and nutrients. This is critical for the health of the ovaries, uterus, and other reproductive tissues.

4. Egg and Sperm Quality: Dehydration may impact egg and sperm quality. Hydration promotes the growth and maturity of these reproductive cells, increasing the likelihood of fertilization success.

5. Detoxification: Adequate hydration promotes the body's natural detoxification processes, assisting in removing toxins and waste products that may interfere with reproductive health.

6. Lubrication and Comfort: Keeping hydrated might help keep you comfortable during intercourse. Inadequate hydration may cause vaginal dryness, making intercourse uncomfortable and possibly decreasing sperm motility.

Techniques for Staying Hydrated

Achieving and maintaining optimal hydration is simple but requires persistent work. Here are some tips to help you remain hydrated:

1. Drink Water regularly: Make it a habit to drink Water throughout the day. To make things easier, bring a reusable water bottle with you.

2. Examine Your Urine: Take note of the colour of your urine. Light yellow or light straw-coloured urine indicates adequate hydration. Dehydration may be indicated by dark yellow or orange urine.

3. Establish Hydration Goals: Aim to drink eight 8-ounce glasses of Water daily (the "8x8" rule) or the quantity your healthcare physician prescribes, depending on your specific requirements.

4. Pay Attention to Your Body: Thirst is your body's method of alerting you to hydration. Please don't ignore it; drink Water when you're thirsty.

5. Consume Hydrating Foods: Include high-water-content foods, such as fruits (e.g., watermelon, oranges) and vegetables (e.g., cucumbers, lettuce).

6. Be Aware of Fluid Loss: Activities such as exercise, hot weather, and sickness may all cause an increase in fluid loss. Keep an extra eye on your hydration during these times.

7. Limit Dehydrating Beverages: Limit your intake of dehydrating beverages such as caffeinated and alcoholic beverages. If you do ingest them, be sure to drink plenty of Water.

8. Herbal teas and infusions help you stay hydrated while providing extra health advantages. Consider chamomile, mint, or red raspberry leaf tea as alternatives.

9. Consult a Healthcare expert: If you have particular concerns about hydration or underlying medical issues that impair fluid balance, get specialized advice from a healthcare expert.

Remember that staying hydrated is a simple yet effective way to promote your reproductive health and fertility. Making Water a priority helps your reproductive system operate correctly and increases your chances of having a healthy pregnancy.

Chapter 3:

3.0 Fertility-Boosting Superfoods

3.1 Exploring Fertility-Boosting Superfoods

Superfoods are nutrient-dense, powerhouse foods that provide a variety of health advantages, including reproductive health and fertility assistance. This chapter will examine fertility-boosting superfoods that may help you conceive and support overall reproductive health.

1. Leafy Greens: Leafy greens, such as spinach, kale, and Swiss chard, are high in folate, a B vitamin essential for embryonic growth. Folate promotes normal cell division and lowers the chance of neural tube abnormalities in the developing baby.

2. Berries: Blueberries, strawberries, and raspberries are high in antioxidants, vitamins, and fibre. These substances aid in the reduction of inflammation, the preservation of egg quality, and the regulation of blood sugar levels.

3. Avocado: Avocado is a nutrient-dense fruit high in monounsaturated fats essential for hormone synthesis and balance. It also contains vitamin E, which may improve the quality of sperm and eggs.

4. Fatty Fish: Fatty fish such as salmon, mackerel, and sardines are high in omega-3 fatty acids. Omega-3 fatty acids decrease inflammation, Help regulate hormones and increase egg quality.

5. Nuts and Seeds: Almonds, walnuts, flaxseeds, and chia seeds are high in healthy fats, fibre, and fertility-boosting minerals such as zinc and selenium. These nuts and seeds help to maintain hormonal balance and reproductive health.

6. Legumes: Plant-based protein, fibre, and folate are abundant in lentils, chickpeas, and black beans. They aid in blood sugar stabilization and supply vital nutrients for reproductive health.

7. Whole Grains: Whole grains such as quinoa, brown rice, and oats are high in complex carbs and fibre. They help to keep blood sugar levels constant and give continuous energy throughout the day.

8. Eggs: Eggs give protein and critical nutrients like choline, which is necessary for embryonic brain development.

9 Dairy or Dairy substitutes: Dairy products and fortified dairy substitutes, such as almond or soy milk, provide calcium and vitamin D, which are essential for bone health and hormone balance.

10 Pomegranate: Pomegranate contains antioxidants that may increase uterine blood flow, thereby improving embryo implantation.

11 Brazil Nuts: These nuts are high in selenium, a mineral that promotes the health and function of sperm.

12 Red Raspberry Leaf: Red raspberry leaf tea tones the uterus and may help with reproductive health.

13. Maca Root: Maca root is an adaptogen that may aid in hormone regulation and fertility.

14. Bee Pollen: Bee pollen contains vitamins, minerals, and amino acids, which may help with reproductive health.

15. Turmeric: Curcumin, an anti-inflammatory substance found in turmeric, may benefit reproductive health.

16. Ginger: Ginger contains anti-inflammatory characteristics and may help with blood circulation, which may help with fertility.

Including these fertility-enhancing superfoods in your diet may be a tasty and proactive strategy to improve your reproductive health. Remember that a well-balanced diet high in nutrient-dense foods is essential to your reproductive quest. Consult a healthcare physician or a qualified dietician for individualized advice based on your specific requirements and objectives.

3.2 Adding Leafy Greens and Vegetables

Leafy greens and vegetables are nutrient-dense foods that are good for your general health and Help with fertility and reproductive health. Here, we look at how to integrate these fertility-boosting items into your diet and some tasty dishes to get you started.

1. Swiss chard

Spinach and Feta Stuffed Chicken Breast Recipe

Ingredients:

- Two skinless, boneless chicken breasts
- 1 cup spinach leaves, fresh
- ¼ cup feta cheese, crumbled
- One minced garlic clove
- Season with salt and pepper to taste.
- Cooking with olive oil

Instructions

Preheat the oven to 375 degrees Fahrenheit (190 degrees Celsius).

Create a pocket in each chicken breast by gently slicing through the middle horizontally, allowing for filling.

Combine the fresh spinach, feta cheese, minced Garlic, salt, and pepper in a mixing bowl.
Stuff each chicken breast with the spinach-feta mixture.

In an oven-safe skillet over medium-high heat, heat the olive oil. Sear the chicken breasts for around 2-3 minutes on each side.

Place the pan in the oven for 20-25 minutes or until the chicken is cooked.

2. Kale

Salad with Kale and Quinoa

Ingredients:

- 2 cups kale leaves, chopped
- 1 cup quinoa, cooked
- A quarter cup of dried cranberries
- ¼ cup almonds, chopped
- Dressing: lemon vinaigrette

To soften the kale, massage it with olive oil and a touch of salt.

Combine the kale, cooked quinoa, dried cranberries, and chopped almonds in a mixing dish.

Toss with the lemon vinaigrette dressing to mix.

3. Broccoli

Broccoli with Parmesan, Roasted
Ingredients:

- 2 cups florets broccoli
- Two teaspoons of olive oil
- Two teaspoons of grated Parmesan cheese
- Season with salt and pepper to taste.
- Optional garnish: lemon zest

Preheat the oven to 425 degrees Fahrenheit (220 degrees Celsius).

Season the broccoli florets with salt and pepper.

On a baking sheet, arrange the broccoli in a single layer.

Roast the broccoli for 20-25 minutes or until soft and slightly crunchy.

Before serving, top with grated Parmesan cheese and lemon zest.

4. Brussels Sprouts

Balsamic Glazed Brussels Sprouts Recipe
Ingredients:

- 2 cups trimmed and halved Brussels sprouts
- Two teaspoons of balsamic vinegar
- One teaspoon of honey
- One minced garlic clove
- Season with salt and pepper to taste.

Preheat the oven to 400 degrees Fahrenheit (200 degrees Celsius).

Mix the balsamic vinegar, honey, minced Garlic, salt, and pepper in a bowl.

Toss the Brussels sprouts with the balsamic dressing. Roast on a baking sheet for 20-25 minutes or until caramelized and soft.

Including leafy greens and vegetables in your diet may be beneficial and tasty. These dishes provide a delicious way to enjoy fertility-boosting meals while supporting your reproductive health. Feel free to add your favourite ingredients and tastes to make them your own.

3.3 Harnessing Berries and Fruits' Power

Berries and fruits are delicious and contain many minerals and antioxidants that may dramatically improve your fertility and general reproductive health. In this chapter, we will look at how to harness the power of these natural riches and present tasty recipes for incorporating them into your everyday diet.

1. Fruits and berries

Berries are high in antioxidants, vitamins, and fibre and include blueberries, strawberries, raspberries, and blackberries. These characteristics make them perfect for improving fertility and reproductive health.

Berry Bliss Smoothie Recipe

Ingredients:

- 1 cup berries (blueberries, strawberries, and raspberries)
- A half banana
- A half-cup of Greek yoghurt
- One teaspoon of honey
- 14 cup almond milk

Blend till smooth the mixed berries, banana, Greek yoghurt, honey, and almond milk.

Pour the smoothie into a glass and serve for breakfast or as a nutritious snack.

2. Citrus Fruits

Citrus fruits, such as oranges, grapefruits, and lemons, are high in vitamin C, which is believed to help with ovulation and sperm function.

Citrus Salad with Mint Dressing Recipe

Ingredients:

- Citrus fruit mixture (oranges, grapefruits, and lemons)
- Mint leaves, fresh
- Honey,
- A grain of salt

Arrange the citrus oranges on a plate after peeling and slicing them.

To make a refreshing dressing, combine finely chopped fresh mint leaves, honey, and a touch of salt in a separate dish.

Serve with the sauce drizzled over the citrus segments.

3. Avocado

Avocado is a fertility-friendly fruit that contains monounsaturated fats and vitamin E, all necessary for hormone synthesis and reproductive health.

Avocado and Mango Salsa Recipe

Ingredients:

- 1 chopped ripe avocado
- 1 diced ripe mango
- ¼ cup coarsely chopped red onion
- Lime juice, chopped cilantro leaves
- Season with salt and pepper to taste.

Combine the diced avocado, mango, red onion, and cilantro in a mixing dish.

Season with salt and pepper after squeezing fresh lime juice over the mixture.

Mix thoroughly and serve over grilled chicken or fish like a salsa.

4. Pomegranate

Pomegranate is high in antioxidants and has been linked to increased uterine blood flow, which may aid in embryo implantation.

Pomegranate Power Smoothie Recipe

Ingredients:

- Pomegranate seeds, ½ cup
- A half-cup of Greek yoghurt
- One banana
- ½ cup spinach leaves (for extra nutrition)
- (Optional) honey drizzle

Smoothly combine the pomegranate seeds, Greek yoghurt, banana, spinach, and honey.

Pour the pomegranate smoothie into a glass and enjoy the fertility-boosting benefits.

3.4 Fertility Nuts, Seeds, and Healthy Fats

Nuts, seeds, and healthy fats are fertility boosters that provide critical nutrients and promote hormonal balance. In this chapter, we look at the advantages of adding these foods to your diet and offer delightful recipes to help you maximize your fertility-boosting potential.

1. Nuts

Nuts like almonds, walnuts, and pistachios are high in healthy fats, protein, and fertility-boosting minerals like zinc and selenium.

Nutty Trail Mix Recipe

Ingredients:

- ¼ cup almonds
- A half-cup of walnuts
- ¼ cup chopped pistachios
- A quarter cup of dried cranberries
- A quarter cup of dark chocolate chips (optional)
- A dash of sea salt

In a mixing dish, combine all of the ingredients.

Portion into little bags for an easy fertility-boosting snack on the road.

2. Seeds

Flaxseeds, chia seeds, and pumpkin seeds are high in omega-3 fatty acids, fibre, and antioxidants, which help hormonal balance and reproductive health.

Chia Seed Pudding

Ingredients:

- 2 tablespoon chia seeds
- ½ cup almond milk (or your chosen milk)
- ½ teaspoon vanilla extract
- 1 tablespoon honey or maple syrup

- Berries for decoration

Combine the chia seeds, almond milk, vanilla essence, and honey (or maple syrup) in a container.

Refrigerate overnight after thoroughly mixing.
Top with mixed berries in the morning for a nutrient-dense and filling breakfast.

3. Good Fats

Healthy fats, such as those found in avocados, olive oil, and fatty fish, aid in hormone synthesis and balance, which is necessary for fertility.

Grilled Salmon with Avocado Salsa

Ingredients:

- Two salmon fillets
- 2 tablespoon olive oil
- Season with salt and pepper to taste

Avocado salsa:

- One ripe avocado, chopped
- ¼ cup chopped red onion
- 14 cups diced tomato
- Lime juice, fresh cilantro leaves

Season with salt and pepper to taste

Preheat the grill to medium-high heat.

Brush salmon fillets with olive oil and season with salt and pepper.

Grill the salmon on each side for 4-5 minutes or until cooked.

To create the avocado salsa, add the chopped avocado, red onion, tomato, cilantro, lime juice, salt, and pepper in a separate bowl.

Serve the grilled salmon with the avocado salsa on the side.

4. Flaxseeds

Flaxseeds are high in fibre and contain lignans, which may help regulate hormones and increase fertility.

Flaxseed Banana Muffins

Ingredients:

- 1 cup whole wheat flour
- ½ cup ground flaxseeds
- One teaspoon of baking soda
- ½ teaspoon cinnamon
- Two ripe bananas, mashed
- ¼ cup honey or maple syrup

- ¼ cup Greek yogurt
- ¼ cup almond milk
- One egg
- One teaspoon of vanilla extract

Preheat the oven to 350°F (175°C) and line a muffin pan with paper liners.

Combine the whole wheat flour, ground flaxseeds, baking soda, and cinnamon in a mixing dish.

Combine the mashed bananas, honey (or maple syrup), Greek yoghurt, almond milk, egg, and vanilla extract in a separate dish.

Stir in the wet ingredients until just mixed.
Bake for 18-20 minutes or until a toothpick inserted comes out clean.

Chapter 4:

4.0 Protein-Rich Recipes for Reproductive Health

4.1 Understanding Protein's Role in Fertility

Protein is an essential macronutrient that affects fertility and reproductive health. In this chapter, we'll look at the significance of protein and how it may help you conceive and have a healthy pregnancy.

1. Protein and Hormone Regulation

Proteins are required for hormone synthesis and control, and hormones play essential roles in the reproductive process. Proteins, for example, are involved in producing and releasing hormones such as estrogen, progesterone, and luteinizing hormone (LH), all essential for menstrual cycle management, ovulation, and implantation.

2. Egg and Sperm Health

Proteins are essential for forming and maintaining healthy eggs in women and sperm in males. They ensure that these reproductive cells receive the nutrition and structural components for successful fertilization. Inadequate protein consumption may result in lower egg and sperm quality.

3. Body Composition and Fertility

Maintaining a healthy body composition, which includes an optimal amount of muscle and a balanced body fat proportion, is essential for fertility. Protein aids in muscle mass preservation and overall body composition. Excessive or inadequate protein consumption in women might impact menstrual regularity and ovulation.

4. Control of Blood Sugar

Protein may help maintain blood sugar levels, essential for hormonal balance. Blood sugar fluctuations may harm fertility, particularly in disorders like polycystic ovarian syndrome (PCOS), where insulin resistance is widespread. A high-protein diet may help with blood sugar regulation.

5. Reproductive Tissue Health

Proteins are the building components for many tissues, including those in the reproductive system. They aid in developing, healing, and maintaining the uterus, ovaries, and testes. Adequate protein intake is critical for the health and function of these reproductive organs.

6. Immune System Support

A healthy immune system is vital for general health and fertility. Proteins assist the immune system by defending the body against infections and creating a healthy environment for conception and pregnancy.

7. Fertility Protein Sources

Consider including the following protein-rich foods into your diet to get the advantages of protein for fertility: Chicken, turkey, and thin cuts of beef or hog are all lean meats.

- **Fish:** Fatty fish such as salmon, mackerel, and sardines are high in protein and omega-3 fatty acids.
- **Eggs:** A good source of protein and other nutrients.
- **Dairy or Dairy Alternatives:** Protein and calcium are provided through Greek yoghurt, cottage cheese, and fortified dairy substitutes.
- Lentils, chickpeas, black beans, and edamame are great plant-based protein sources.
- Almonds, walnuts, chia seeds, and flaxseeds are high in protein and good fats.
- Tofu and Tempeh are flexible plant-based protein sources.

Protein Consumption Must Be Balanced

It's critical to establish a balance when it comes to protein consumption. Excessive protein consumption may be harmful to fertility, as can inadequate intake. Aim for a balanced diet that contains a range of protein sources to ensure that you achieve your nutritional requirements. Consultation with a healthcare physician or certified dietitian may assist you in determining the optimal protein consumption for your unique condition and dietary choices. A balanced, protein-rich diet may help you improve your fertility and reproductive health.

4.2 Lean Meat and Poultry Dishes

Incorporating lean meats and poultry into your diet may give essential protein and minerals that promote fertility. Here are some tasty and fertility-friendly meals to help you enjoy these protein-rich alternatives.

1. Grilled chicken breast with Mediterranean Quinoa Salad

Ingredients:

- Two boneless, skinless chicken breasts
- 1 cup quinoa
- 2 cups water or chicken broth

- One cucumber, diced
- 1 cup cherry tomatoes, halved
- ¼ cup red onion, finely chopped Kalamata olives, pitted and sliced Feta cheese, crumbled
- Olive oil, fresh parsley
- Lemon juice
- Season with salt and pepper to taste

Instructions:

Season the chicken breasts with salt, pepper, and olive oil. Grill till done.

Rinse the quinoa under cool Water. Combine the quinoa with the Water or chicken stock in a saucepan. Bring to a boil, then lower to a low heat, cover, and let to cook for 15-20 minutes, or until the quinoa is tender and the Water has been absorbed.

Allow the quinoa to cool before fluffing it with a fork. Combine the quinoa, cucumber, cherry tomatoes, red onion, olives, and feta cheese in a large mixing bowl.

Mix the olive oil, lemon juice, salt, and pepper in a small bowl to make the dressing.

Toss the salad with the dressing.

Topped with fresh parsley, serve the grilled chicken on top of the Mediterranean quinoa salad.

2. Balsamic Glazed Salmon

Ingredients:

- Two salmon fillets
- 2 tablespoon olive oil
- Season with salt and pepper to taste
- Balsamic glaze (store-bought or handmade using balsamic vinegar and honey)

Instructions:

Preheat the oven to 375°F (190°C).

Season the salmon fillets with salt and pepper.

In an oven-safe skillet, heat the olive oil over medium-high heat.

Sear salmon fillets for 2-3 minutes on each side.
Bake for 10-12 minutes in a preheated oven.

Drizzle the balsamic glaze over the fish shortly before serving.

3. Stuffed bell peppers with turkey and quinoa

Ingredients:

- Four bell peppers, any colour
- ½ cup quinoa
- 1 cup water or chicken broth
- 1 pound lean ground turkey
- One onion, finely chopped
- One can of diced tomatoes (14 oz)
- 1 cup spinach, chopped Italian seasoning
- Season with salt and pepper to taste
- Optional: shredded mozzarella cheese

Instructions:

Preheat the oven to 350°F (175°C).

Remove the tops of the bell peppers and remove the seeds and membranes.

Rinse the quinoa under cool Water. Combine the quinoa with the Water or chicken stock in a saucepan. Bring to a boil, then lower to a low heat, cover, and let to cook for 15-20 minutes, or until the quinoa is tender and the Water has been absorbed.

Brown the ground turkey in a pan over medium heat. Cook until the onion is transparent.

Stir in the diced tomatoes, spinach, cooked quinoa, Italian seasoning, salt, and pepper. Cook for a couple more minutes.

Stuff the bell peppers with the turkey-quinoa mixture.

Place the filled bell peppers in a baking dish, cover with foil, and bake for 30-35 minutes or until the peppers are soft.

Sprinkle shredded mozzarella cheese on top of each pepper during the final 10 minutes of baking.

Plant-Based Protein Substitutes

You're in luck if you want to enhance your fertility using plant-based protein sources. Plant-based proteins may deliver the vital nutrients your body needs for reproductive health while providing various tastes and textures. Here are some plant-based protein options and dishes to include in your fertility-friendly diet:

1. Lentils

Lentils are a flexible source of plant-based protein high in folate and iron, crucial for fertility.

Lentil and Vegetable Stir-Fry

Ingredients:

- 1 cup dry green or brown lentils
- Vegetables (bell peppers, broccoli, carrots, snow peas)

- Minced Garlic and ginger
- Soy sauce (low sodium) or tamari Sesame oil
- Optional red pepper flakes
- Brown rice or quinoa cooked (optional, for serving)

Set aside the lentils after cooking them according to package directions.

Heat sesame oil in a big pan or wok over medium-high heat.

Stir in the minced Garlic and ginger for a minute.

Cook until the veggies are slightly soft, about 5 minutes.

Add the cooked lentils and a dash of low-sodium soy sauce or tamari to taste.

If desired, season with red pepper flakes.

For a balanced dinner, serve over brown rice or quinoa.

2. fava beans

Chickpeas are high in protein, fibre, and folate, which may help fertility.

Curry with Chickpeas and Spinach

Ingredients:

- One can of chickpeas, washed and drained
- One finely chopped onion, Garlic and ginger, minced
- One tin chopped tomatoes
- Spinach stems
- Curry powder or curry paste
- Coconut cream
- Extra virgin olive oil
- Season with salt and pepper to taste.
- Basmati rice, cooked (optional for serving)

In a large skillet over medium heat, heat the olive oil.

Mix in the onion, Garlic, and ginger. Sauté the onion until it is transparent.

Stir in the curry powder or paste (tune the spiciness to your liking).

Combine chopped tomatoes, chickpeas, and a can of coconut milk in a mixing bowl.

Simmer, stirring periodically, for 10-15 minutes.

Cook until the spinach leaves are wilted.

Season with salt and pepper to taste.

If preferred, serve over cooked basmati rice.

3. Tofu

Tofu is an excellent plant-based protein source that can be utilized in several ways.

Stir-fry with Tofu and Vegetables

Ingredients:

- Tofu that has been diced and squeezed to remove extra Water
- Vegetable mixture (bell peppers, broccoli, snap peas, carrots)
- Soy sauce with low sodium or teriyaki sauce
- Minced Garlic and ginger
- Sesame oil or olive oil
- Brown rice or quinoa cooked (optional, for serving)

In a large skillet or wok, heat the oil over medium-high heat.

Stir in the minced Garlic and ginger for a minute.

Cook until the cubed tofu is browned on both sides.

Stir in the mixed veggies until they are tender-crisp.

Drizzle the tofu and vegetables with low-sodium soy sauce or teriyaki sauce.

If preferred, serve over cooked brown rice or quinoa.

4. Quinoa

Quinoa is a complete protein which includes all necessary amino acids, making it an excellent plant-based alternative for fertility.

Quinoa Salad with Roasted Vegetables Recipe

Ingredients:

- 1 cup cooked quinoa
- Vegetables assorted (zucchini, bell peppers, cherry tomatoes, red onion)
- Balsamic vinegar, olive oil
- chopped fresh basil leaves
- Season with salt and pepper to taste.

Cook quinoa according to package directions after rinsing it under cool Water.

Preheat the oven to 425 degrees Fahrenheit (220 degrees Celsius).

Toss the veggies in a bowl with olive oil, balsamic vinegar, salt, and pepper.

Bake the veggies until soft and slightly browned.

Combine the cooked quinoa, roasted veggies, and fresh basil in a large mixing basin.

If preferred, drizzle with more olive oil and balsamic vinegar.

These plant-based protein substitutes and dishes provide a nutritional and fertility-friendly option to satisfy your protein requirements while enjoying a range of tastes and textures. Incorporate these foods into your diet to enhance your reproductive health.

4.4 Protein in Combination with Essential Nutrients

To improve fertility, you must concentrate on protein consumption and mix it with nutrients crucial for reproductive health. Here are some fertility-friendly protein and nutrient combinations, as well as dishes that highlight these pairings:

1. Folate and protein

In the early stages of pregnancy, folate is required for proper cell division and neural tube development. Combining protein-rich diets with folate-rich components will help you become more fertile.

Salmon with Asparagus Recipe

Salmon is a high-protein food high in omega-3 fatty acids, whereas asparagus is high in folate.

Ingredients:

- Fillets of salmon
- Asparagus spears, fresh
- Extra virgin olive oil
- Juice of lemon
- Minced garlic cloves
- Season with salt and pepper to taste.

Preheat the oven to 375 degrees Fahrenheit (190 degrees Celsius).

On a baking sheet, arrange the salmon fillets and asparagus.

Drizzle with lemon juice and olive oil.

Sprinkle with minced Garlic, salt, and pepper.

Bake the salmon for 15-20 minutes or until it flakes easily with a fork.

2. Iron and protein

Iron is required for healthy blood and the prevention of anaemia. Combining protein with iron-rich meals will help ensure you receive enough of this vital vitamin.

Curry with Spinach and Lentils

Spinach contains iron, while lentils provide plant-based protein.

Ingredients:

- 1 cup green or brown lentils, dry
- Spinach leaves, chopped
- Minced onion, Garlic, and ginger
- Diced canned tomatoes
- Coconut cream
- Spices for curry (turmeric, cumin, coriander, garam masala)
- Extra virgin olive oil
- Season with salt and pepper to taste.
- Brown rice, cooked (optional for serving)

Set aside the lentils after cooking them according to package directions.

Warm the olive oil in a large pan over medium heat.

Mix in the onion, Garlic, and ginger. Cook until fragrant.

Cook for a minute after adding the curry spices.

Combine canned diced tomatoes, lentils, and chopped spinach in a mixing bowl.

Pour in the coconut milk and cook until the spinach wilts and everything is hot.

Season with salt and pepper to taste.

If preferred, serve over cooked brown rice.

3. Antioxidants and Protein

Antioxidants aid in the protection of reproductive cells from oxidative damage, which may impair fertility. Combining protein with antioxidant-rich foods may offer a dietary boost beneficial to fertility.

Parfait with Berries and Greek Yogurt

Greek yoghurt is high in protein, while berries are high in antioxidants.

Ingredients:

- Yoghurt from Greece
- Berries (strawberries, blueberries, and raspberries)
- Optional sweetener: honey or maple syrup
- Optional granola (for extra texture)

Layer Greek yoghurt and mixed berries in a glass or dish.

If preferred, drizzle with honey or maple syrup for sweetness.

For extra crunch, sprinkle with granola.

Combining protein with these essential nutrients makes creating balanced and healthy meals that promote fertility possible. Experiment with these combinations and recipes to make tasty and fertility-friendly foods personalized to your tastes.

Chapter 5

5.0 Carbohydrates and Fertility: Finding the Right Balance

5.1 The Effect of Carbohydrates on Insulin Levels

The link between carbs and insulin levels is critical for fertility and reproductive health. Insulin, a pancreatic hormone, is essential in maintaining blood sugar levels, but its levels may also impact other hormonal processes that affect fertility.

Here's how carbohydrates affect insulin levels and what its implications are for your reproductive health:

1. Blood Sugar and Carbohydrates

During digestion, carbohydrates are broken down into glucose (sugar) and taken into circulation. The kind and amount of carbs you eat may significantly impact your blood sugar levels.

2. Carbohydrates: Simple vs. Complex

Simple carbohydrate sources include sugar, white bread, and processed snacks. They swiftly elevate blood sugar levels, causing insulin to be released.

Complex carbohydrate foods include entire grains, legumes, vegetables, and fruits. They digest slowly, resulting in a more gradual rise in blood sugar and a more regulated insulin response.

3. Hormone and Insulin Regulation

Insulin's principal function is to assist cells in absorbing glucose from the circulation and using it for energy. However, insulin also has a secondary role in the regulation of other hormones, particularly those involved in reproduction:

- Insulin may affect sex hormone levels, such as estrogen and testosterone, essential for reproductive health. High insulin levels may cause hormonal abnormalities, possibly impacting ovulation and sperm production.

- PCOS (Polycystic Ovary Syndrome): PCOS is a prevalent hormonal condition that affects women of reproductive age. It is often connected with insulin resistance, a condition in which the body's cells do not react appropriately to insulin. This might result in high insulin levels, which can cause irregular menstrual periods and reproductive issues.

4. Carbohydrate Balance for Fertility

It is essential to balance your carbohydrate consumption to manage insulin levels and maintain fertility:

Select Complex Carbohydrates: Whole grains, lentils, and fibrous vegetables provide consistent energy without producing blood sugar spikes.

Limit Simple Sugars: Sugary drinks, candy, and processed meals with added sugars should be avoided since they might cause fast insulin release.

Fibre and Protein: Include fibre-rich foods and protein sources daily. Fibre inhibits glucose absorption, whereas protein helps to keep blood sugar levels stable.

Moderation: Watch your portion sizes and total carbohydrate consumption. Because everyone's carbohydrate requirements differ, it's essential to discover a balance that works for you.

Consult a Healthcare Professional: If you have questions about insulin levels, blood sugar management, or disorders like PCOS, speak with your doctor or a qualified dietitian. They may provide specialized advice and suggestions based on your specific requirements.

A well-rounded diet that balances carbohydrate consumption and manages insulin levels may contribute to greater reproductive health and support your fertility objectives.

5.2 Selecting the Correct Carbohydrates

Choosing the proper carbs may significantly influence your fertility and reproductive health. Focusing on quality and making good choices regarding carbs may help balance blood sugar levels, regulate hormones, and support your reproductive objectives. Here's how to choose the best carbohydrates:

1. Adopt Whole Grains

Whole grains are high in complex carbs, fibre, vitamins, and minerals. They give prolonged energy and assist in reducing blood sugar increases. Include the following whole grains in your diet:

- Brown rice is a healthy alternative to white rice, high in fibre and essential minerals.
- Quinoa is a complete protein that has a subtle, nutty taste.
- **Oatmeal:** High in fibre and recognized for its heart-healthy properties.
- **Whole wheat:** For more fibre, use whole wheat bread, pasta, and flour.

2. Make Fiber-Rich Foods a Priority

Fibre-rich meals delay glucose absorption, supporting stable blood sugar levels. They also promote intestinal health and may assist with weight control, all necessary for fertility. Include the following fibre-rich options:

Legumes: Beans, lentils, and chickpeas are high in fibre and plant-based protein.

Fruits: To increase fibre consumption, choose whole fruits with skin, such as apples, pears, and berries.

Vegetables: Leafy greens, broccoli, and carrots are fibre-rich vegetables for your diet.

3. Restrict Added Sugars

Excessive added sugars may cause fast blood sugar increases and have a detrimental impact on fertility. Be wary of sugary meals and drinks like soda, candy, pastries, and cereals. Examine food labels and try to limit your intake of these things.

4. Select Low-Glycemic Carbohydrates

The glycemic index (GI) of carbohydrates evaluates how rapidly they boost blood sugar levels. Low GI foods digest more slowly, producing more stable blood sugar levels. Choose low-GI carbs such as:

- **Sweet potatoes:** A nutrient-dense option with a slow release of energy.
- Whole-grain pasta is preferred over regular pasta because of its lower GI and increased fibre content.
- Berries are low in sugar and abundant in antioxidants, making them an ideal low-GI snack.

5. Carbohydrates should be balanced with protein and healthy fats.

Combining carbs with protein and healthy fats may help to normalize blood sugar levels and promote fertility. As an example:

- **Greek yoghurt with berries:** Combines berries' carbs with yoghurt's protein and probiotics.

- **Avocado toast:** Avocado toast provides healthful fats to balance out the carbohydrates in whole-grain bread.
- **Hummus with vegetables:** Provides fibre-rich vegetables, protein, and healthy fats from hummus.

6. Keep an eye on portion sizes

While picking the proper carbs is essential, portion control also plays a part in blood sugar management. Remember portion proportions to prevent overconsumption, which may contribute to excess calorie intake and weight gain.

5.3 Whole Grains and Legumes and Their Health Benefits

Whole grains and legumes are nutritional powerhouses that may help boost fertility and reproductive health. They are high in critical nutrients and provide a variety of advantages that may improve your overall health. Here's a rundown of the benefits of whole grains and legumes:

1. Grain Whole:

Fiber-Rich Whole Grains: Whole grains including brown rice, quinoa, and whole wheat are high in fibre. Fiber aids in the regulation of blood sugar levels, the prevention of insulin spikes, and the maintenance of consistent energy levels throughout the day. It also promotes good digestion and may assist with weight management, essential for fertility.

Whole grains are high in vitamins (B vitamins, including folate) and minerals (iron, magnesium, and zinc) necessary for reproductive health. Folate, in particular, is essential for preventing birth abnormalities and maintaining a healthy pregnancy.

Heart Health: Eating whole grains has been linked to a lower risk of heart disease. A robust cardiovascular system is essential for general health, including reproductive health.

Antioxidants: Antioxidants are included in many whole grains and help protect cells from oxidative damage. This is especially crucial for sperm and egg quality.

2. Legumes:

Plant-Based Protein: Legumes, such as beans, lentils, and chickpeas, are high in plant-based protein. Protein is required for cell development, repair, hormone synthesis, and reproductive health.

Folate Content: Legumes are high in folate, which is necessary to prevent neural tube abnormalities in the early stages of pregnancy. Women who are attempting to conceive must consume enough folate.

Fibre and Blood Sugar Control: The fibre content of legumes aids in the stabilization of blood sugar levels and the reduction of insulin surges. This may help with hormonal balance, particularly for those with polycystic ovarian syndrome (PCOS) or insulin resistance.

Iron & Nutrient Density: Legumes include iron, an essential mineral for keeping healthy blood and avoiding anaemia. During pregnancy, when blood volume rises, iron is incredibly vital.

Low in Saturated Fat: Legumes are naturally expected in saturated fat, so they are a heart-healthy option. A robust cardiovascular system benefits reproductive health in general.

Adding Whole Grains and Legumes to Your Diet:

- Quinoa may make grain bowls, salads, or a side dish. Quinoa has all of the essential amino acids.

- **Brown Rice:** Replace white rice in your meals with brown rice for more fibre and minerals.

- **Whole Wheat**: To improve your consumption of whole grains, use whole wheat pasta, bread, and flour for baking.

- Adding kidney beans, black beans, and chickpeas may benefit from soups, stews, salads, and pasta meals.

- **Lentils:** Use lentils to make substantial soups and stews or as a meat alternative in dishes like lentil burgers or tacos.

- **Hummus:** Serve as a dip or spread over whole wheat crackers or veggies for a nutritious snack.

Including a variety of whole grains and legumes in your diet may give your body the nutrients it needs for fertility and reproductive health. They provide a well-balanced blend of fibre, protein, vitamins, and minerals that benefit your overall health and increase your chances of conceiving and keeping a healthy pregnancy.

5.4 Sustained Energy and Fertility Support Recipes

Maintaining consistent energy levels while maintaining your fertility is critical for overall health. To help you reach both objectives, these recipes use nutrient-dense foods such as whole grains, legumes, and healthy fats. These recipes are not only tasty, but they are also beneficial to reproductive health:

Salad with Quinoa and Black Beans

Ingredients:

- 1 cup cooked quinoa
- 2 cups water/vegetable broth
- One can of black beans, washed and drained
- 1 cup fresh or frozen corn kernels
- Halved cherry tomatoes
- Finely sliced red onion
- Fresh cilantro, avocado, and olive oil cubed
- Juice of lime
- Season with salt and pepper to taste.

Instructions:

Rinse the quinoa with cool Water. Combine quinoa and water or vegetable broth in a saucepan. Bring to a boil, lower to low heat, cover, and cook for 15-20 minutes or until the quinoa is tender and the liquid has been absorbed. Allow it to cool.

Combine the cooked quinoa, black beans, corn, cherry tomatoes, red onion, cilantro, and avocado in a large mixing basin.

Mix the olive oil, lime juice, salt, and pepper in a separate bowl to make the dressing.

Drizzle the dressing over the salad and gently mix to combine. Chill before serving.

2. Stir-fry of Lentils and Vegetables

Ingredients:

- 1 cup green or brown lentils, dry
- Vegetable mixture (bell peppers, broccoli, carrots, snow peas)
- Minced Garlic and ginger
- Soy sauce with low sodium or teriyaki sauce
- Sesame seed oil
- Extra virgin olive oil
- Brown rice or quinoa cooked (optional, for serving)

Instructions:

Set aside the lentils after cooking them according to package directions.

Warm the olive oil in a big pan or wok over medium-high heat.

Stir in the minced Garlic and ginger for a minute.

Cook until the veggies are slightly soft, about 5 minutes.

Mix well with the cooked lentils and a dab of low-sodium soy or teriyaki sauce.

For a full meal, serve overcooked brown rice or quinoa.

3. Parfait with Berries and Greek Yogurt

Ingredients:

- Yoghurt from Greece
- Berries (strawberries, blueberries, and raspberries)
- Optional sweetener: honey or maple syrup
- Optional granola (for extra texture)

Instructions:

Layer Greek yoghurt and mixed berries in a glass or dish.

If preferred, drizzle with honey or maple syrup for sweetness.

For extra crunch, sprinkle with granola.

These recipes use nutrient-dense foods to give prolonged energy and reproductive assistance. Whole grains, legumes, healthy fats, and antioxidants are among them, and they all contribute to general reproductive health and well-being. Consume these foods as part of a well-balanced diet to increase your chances of conceiving and having a healthy pregnancy.

Chapter 6

6.0 Cooking for Hormonal Balance,

6.1 Ingredients that balance hormones

Hormone balance is critical for reproductive health and fertility. Certain foods in your diet may influence hormone regulation. Here are some hormone-balancing items you may include in your meals to help with fertility:

1. Fatty Acids Omega-3

Omega-3 fatty acids, notably EPA and DHA (docosahexaenoic acid), are required for hormone synthesis and control. They are also anti-inflammatory, which may help with general health and fertility.
Fatty fish (salmon, mackerel, sardines), flaxseeds, chia seeds, and walnuts are good sources.

2. Greens with a lot of leaves

Folate, a B vitamin essential for hormone production and control, is abundant in leafy green vegetables. Folate is crucial during the first trimester of pregnancy to avoid neural tube abnormalities.
Spinach, kale, Swiss chard, broccoli, and collard greens are good sources.

3. Vegetables with a high cruciferous content

Compounds found in cruciferous vegetables, such as indole-3-carbinol (I3C), may help regulate estrogen levels by stimulating the breakdown of excess estrogen.
Broccoli, cauliflower, Brussels sprouts, kale, and cabbage are good sources.

4. Avocado

Avocado is high in monounsaturated fats, which help in hormone synthesis. It also contains vitamin E, which has been shown to improve fertility.

5. Berries

Berries are high in antioxidants, which aid in the fight against oxidative stress and inflammation, which may interfere with hormonal balance and fertility.
Blueberries, strawberries, and raspberries are good sources.

6. Lentils with beans

Beans and lentils are high in plant-based protein and fibre. They may aid in regulating blood sugar levels and promoting hormone stability.

7. Seeds and nuts

Nuts and seeds include healthful fats as well as critical elements. They may help with hormone production as well as general reproductive health.
Almonds, walnuts, chia seeds, and flaxseeds are good sources.

8. Fish with a lot of fat

Fatty fish, such as salmon and mackerel, supply omega-3 fatty acids and vitamin D. Vitamin D is involved in hormone control and may help with conception.

9. The spice turmeric

Curcumin is found in turmeric, a chemical recognized for its anti-inflammatory qualities. It may aid in reducing inflammation, which may affect hormone balance.

10. Dairy or Dairy Substitutes

Calcium and vitamin D, vital for hormonal health, may be found in dairy products and fortified dairy substitutes.

11. Ginger

Ginger contains anti-inflammatory effects and may aid in the regulation of menstrual cycles, making it useful for women with irregular periods.

12. Lean Protein

Lean protein foods like chicken, turkey, and tofu include amino acids required for hormone production.

6.2 Menstrual Cycle Support Recipes

Eating a well-balanced diet rich in particular nutrients might help support your menstrual cycle and ease symptoms such as cramps, bloating, and mood changes. Here are two dishes that can give essential nutrients while also promoting menstrual health:

Smoothie to Balance Hormones

This smoothie has components high in vitamins, minerals, and antioxidants, which may aid in hormone balance and inflammation reduction.

Ingredients:

- 1 cup spinach or kale (for iron and folate)
- ½ cup berries (to boost antioxidants)
- ½ banana (for potassium and B6)
- 1 tablespoon flaxseeds (for omega-3 fatty acids)
- ½ cup Greek yoghurt (high in calcium and probiotics)
- ½ cup almond milk (or other milk of choice)
- One teaspoon of honey (optional for added sweetness)

Instructions:

In a blender, combine all of the ingredients.

Blend until the mixture is smooth and creamy.

Adjust the sweetness with honey if necessary.

Pour into a glass and serve as a healthy breakfast or snack.

2. Quinoa Anti-Inflammatory Bowl

This quinoa meal is high in anti-inflammatory components, which may help alleviate period pain and maintain hormonal balance.

Ingredients:

- 1 cup cooked quinoa (for fibre, protein, and folate)
- ½ cup chickpeas (for protein and fibre)
- ½ cup cooked broccoli (for fibre and calcium)
- ¼ cup chopped avocado (for potassium and good fats)
- ¼ cup pomegranate seeds (to boost antioxidants)
- 2 tablespoon tahini (for calcium and good fats)
- Lemon juice (for taste)
- Season with salt and pepper to taste.

Instructions:

Cook the quinoa according to package directions and set aside to cool.
Combine cooked quinoa, chickpeas, steamed broccoli, cubed avocado, and pomegranate seeds in a mixing dish.

Drizzle with tahini and lemon juice to finish.

Season to taste with salt and pepper.

Toss everything together until well combined.

Assemble as a filling lunch or supper choice.

6.3 PCOS and Other Hormonal Problems

PCOS and other hormonal disorders may substantially influence fertility and general well-being. While there is no one-size-fits-all approach, adopting educated food and lifestyle choices may aid symptom management and hormonal balance. Here are some broad pointers and suggestions:

1. A well-balanced diet:

Foods with a Low Glycemic Index (GI): Choose complex carbs with a low GI to help manage blood sugar levels and prevent insulin resistance, which is frequent in PCOS.

Meals High in Fiber: Fiber-rich meals such as whole grains, legumes, and vegetables help balance blood sugar and improve digestive health.

Lean Protein: To promote hormone production, include lean protein sources in your meals such as chicken, fish, tofu, and beans.

Avocados, almonds, seeds, and olive oil are all excellent sources of healthy fats that may help with hormonal balance.

Limit Added Sugars: Sugary meals and drinks should be avoided since they might aggravate insulin resistance and hormonal abnormalities.

Fatty fish, flaxseeds, and chia seeds are high in omega-3 fatty acids, which have anti-inflammatory qualities.

Moderate Dairy: Some people with PCOS may benefit from limiting their dairy intake since it might decrease insulin sensitivity. Consider dairy substitutes such as almond milk or lactose-free alternatives.

2. Portion Control and Meal Balance:

Eating frequent, balanced meals and limiting calorie consumption may aid with weight control, which is vital for PCOS treatment.

Consider seeking specialized advice from a licensed dietician who specializes in PCOS.

3. Workout:

Physical exercise regularly may enhance insulin sensitivity and aid with weight control.
Aim for aerobic (like brisk walking) and strength training workouts.
Find things that you like to maintain a consistent workout program.

4. Stress Reduction:

Chronic stress might throw off your hormonal equilibrium. Yoga, meditation, deep breathing, and mindfulness are all stress-reduction strategies.

5. Sleep:

Prioritize quality sleep since insufficient sleep may interfere with hormone control and worsen hormonal disorders.

6. Additions:

Before taking supplements, consult your doctor. However, some women with PCOS may benefit from inositol, vitamin D, and chromium.

7. Routine Check-Ups:

Make frequent appointments with your doctor to assess your hormonal health and discuss treatment choices.

8. Groups of Support:

Joining a support group or seeking counselling may provide emotional support and practical Help for dealing with PCOS or hormonal difficulties.

It's important to note that dealing with PCOS and hormonal disorders frequently necessitates a holistic strategy. Dietary and lifestyle adjustments may help, but everyone's demands are different. Consultation with a healthcare physician or a registered dietitian specializing in hormonal disorders may assist you in developing a customized plan that is suited to your circumstances.

Chapter 7

7.0 Meal Plans, Menus, and Lifestyle Suggestions

7.1 Developing Fertility-Inducing Meal Plans

Day	Meal	Fertility-Boosting Foods
Day 1	Breakfast	Greek yogurt with mixed berries and honey
	Lunch	Whole grain toast with almond butter - Spinach and lentil salad with a lemon-tahini dressing - Quinoa side dish
	Dinner	Baked salmon with asparagus and quinoa

	Snack	Carrot and cucumber sticks with hummus
Day 2	Breakfast	Oatmeal with sliced bananas and walnuts
	Lunch	Chickpea and vegetable stir-fry with brown rice
	Dinner	Grilled chicken breast with broccoli and sweet potatoes
	Snack	Mixed nuts and a small apple
Day 3	Breakfast	-Scrambled eggs with spinach and tomatoes - Whole grain toast
	Lunch	Lentil and vegetable soup with a side salad
	Dinner	Quinoa and black bean stuffed bell peppers

	Snack	Greek yogurt with a drizzle of honey
Day 4	Breakfast	Whole grain pancakes with fresh berries
	Lunch	Tuna salad with mixed greens and olive oil vinaigrette
	Dinner	Baked cod with roasted Brussels sprouts and quinoa
	Snack	Sliced pear with almond butte
Day 5	Breakfast	Smoothie with spinach, banana, chia seeds, and almond milk
	Lunch	Quinoa and chickpea salad with a lemon-tahini dressing
	Dinner	Stir-fried tofu with broccoli and brown rice
	Snack	Mixed berries and a handful of almonds

Day 6	Breakfast	Cottage cheese with pineapple and a sprinkle of flaxseeds
	Lunch	Turkey and avocado wrap with whole wheat tortilla
	Dinner	Grilled shrimp with asparagus and quinoa
	Snack	Celery sticks with peanut butter
Day 7	Breakfast	Scrambled eggs with mushrooms and whole grain toast
	Lunch	Quinoa and vegetable stir-fry with tofu
	Dinner	Baked chicken breast with roasted sweet potatoes and green beans
	Snack	Cottage cheese with sliced strawberries

7.2 Seasonal Menus to Provide Variety

Creating seasonal meals may help you add diversity to your diet while ensuring you get the freshest and most delicious items available all year. Seasonal meals for each of the four seasons are provided below:

Menu for Spring:

Breakfast:

- Smoothie with fresh berries and spinach
- Avocado and poached egg on whole-grain bread

Lunch:

- Salad with spinach and strawberries with balsamic vinaigrette
- Lemon and herb-grilled chicken breast

Dinner:

- Risotto with asparagus and peas
- Salmon baked in a dill and yoghurt sauce
- Artichokes steamed with garlic aioli

Snacks:

- Hummus with cucumber and radishes, Greek yoghurt with honey, and sliced kiwi

Menu for the Summer:

Breakfast:

- Parfait of Greek yoghurt with seasonal fruit and oats

Lunch:
- iced coffee or tea
- Salad Caprese with fresh tomatoes, mozzarella, and basil
- Salad with grilled vegetables and quinoa

Dinner:

- Grilled shrimp skewers with zucchini and summer squash
- Bruschetta with tomato and basil
- Chili-lime butter corn on the cob

Snacks:

- Bites of watermelon with feta cheese
- Peaches, sliced, with a dusting of cinnamon

Menu for the Fall:

Breakfast:

- Oatmeal with pumpkin spice and pecans

Lunch:

- Warm apple cider
- Soup with butternut squash
- Salad of mixed greens with apples, cranberries, and walnuts

Dinner:

- Chicken roasted with root vegetables (carrots, potatoes, and parsnips)
- Acorn squash filled with quinoa
- Brussels sprouts sautéed with bacon and shallots

Snacks:

- Apples baked with cinnamon and topped with Greek yoghurt
- Pumpkin seeds, roasted

Menu for the Winter:

Breakfast:

- Winter spices (cinnamon, nutmeg) and dried cranberries with overnight oats

Lunch:
- Hot herbal tea
- Soup with vegetables and lentils
- Salad with spinach and pomegranate

Dinner:
- Beef stew cooked slowly with carrots and potatoes
- Maple-glazed roasted winter squash
- Mashed potatoes with Garlic

Snacks:

- Pear slices with almond butter
- A handful of mixed nuts and dark chocolate

These seasonal dinners showcase each season's wealth while providing diverse tastes and nutrients. Adapt the recipes to your dietary choices and nutritional requirements, and feel free to use locally produced or seasonal products for an even fresher experience. Keep hydrated with Water or herbal teas, and work with a certified dietitian to create a tailored eating plan based on your health and nutritional objectives.

7.3 Nutritional Supplements and Guidelines

Nutrition is essential for fertility and reproductive health. Specific vitamins, nutritional advice, and a well-balanced diet may help you on your way to conception and a successful pregnancy. Here are some significant suggestions:

1. Folic acid (Folate):

To avoid neural tube abnormalities in early pregnancy, most women of reproductive age should take a daily dose of 400-800 micrograms (mcg) of folic acid.
Leafy greens, fortified cereals, beans, lentils, and citrus fruits are all good sources.

2. Iron:

You may need to take iron supplements if you have iron deficiency anaemia. For tailored advice, speak with a healthcare practitioner.
Lean meats, chicken, fish, fortified cereals, beans, and spinach are all excellent sources of iron.

3. Vitamin D:

If you have low vitamin D levels, consider taking a supplement, mainly if you reside in an area with minimal sunshine.
Fatty fish (salmon, mackerel), fortified dairy products, egg yolks, and sunshine exposure are good sources.

4. Fatty Acids Omega-3:

Some people may benefit from omega-3 supplementation (such as fish oil or algae-based supplements) to help with reproductive health.
Fatty fish, flaxseeds, chia seeds, walnuts, and hemp seeds are all excellent sources.

5. CoQ10 (Coenzyme Q10):

CoQ10 pills may assist women to increase their egg quality. For dose suggestions, speak with your doctor.
CoQ10 is in trace levels in organ meats, seafood, and whole grains.

6. Antioxidants:

Antioxidant supplements (e.g., vitamin C, E) may help battle oxidative stress, affecting fertility.
Berries, citrus fruits, nuts, seeds, and colourful vegetables are all good sources of antioxidants.

7. Multivitamin:

A daily prenatal or multivitamin may assist in addressing nutritional gaps, but it should not be used instead of a well-balanced diet.

Sources of nutrition: Various meals are recommended to guarantee a wide range of nutrients.
Nutritional Recommendations:

Balanced Diet: Make entire grains, lean proteins, healthy fats, and fruits and vegetables a priority.

Fibre: Consume fibre-rich foods such as whole grains, legumes, and veggies to help regulate digestive health and blood sugar.

Hydration: Drink plenty of Water and herbal teas to stay hydrated, and limit caffeine and alcohol intake.

Limit Processed Foods: Limit your consumption of processed and sugary foods, which may harm fertility.

Portion Control: Pay attention to portion sizes to maintain a healthy weight, which is essential for fertility.

Stress Management: To improve reproductive health, use stress-reduction practices such as yoga, meditation, or deep breathing exercises.

Schedule frequent check-ups with a healthcare practitioner to assess your general health and address any particular reproductive problems.

7.4 Fertility Enhancing Lifestyle Practices

Healthy lifestyle choices that enhance reproductive health and general well-being are often associated with increasing fertility. Consider the following critical lifestyle practices:

1. Keep a Healthy Weight:

Both women and men may benefit from achieving and maintaining a healthy weight. Extra body fat might cause hormonal abnormalities.

2. Consume a Well-balanced Diet:

Make a balanced diet with whole grains, lean proteins, healthy fats, and a variety of fruits and vegetables a priority. Nutrient-dense diets provide vitamins and minerals that are needed for reproductive health.

3. Stress Management:

Stress may interfere with hormonal balance and menstrual periods. Meditation, yoga, deep breathing exercises, and mindfulness are all stress-reduction practices.

4. Exercise on a regular basis:

Maintain a healthy weight and general well-being by engaging in frequent physical exercise. Excessive or severe activity, on the other hand, might have a detrimental influence on fertility in certain situations.

5. Get Enough Sleep:

Prioritize quality sleep since insufficient sleep may interfere with hormone control and reproductive health. Limit your intake of alcohol and caffeine:

Excessive intake of alcohol and caffeine might have a detrimental influence on fertility. Limit your consumption and consider removing or minimizing your exposure to these chemicals.

7. Quit Smoking:

Both men and women may be harmed by Smoking. If you smoke, get HelpHelp quitting.

8. Avoid Potentially Harmful Environmental Exposures:

Reduce exposure to environmental toxins and pollutants such as chemicals, pesticides, and radiation, which may impact reproductive health.

9. Keep Hydrated:

Drink enough Water to improve your general health and reproductive function.

10. Practice Safe Sex: - By practising safe sex, you may protect yourself from sexually transmitted diseases (STIs). If left untreated, several STIs might cause reproductive issues.

11. Monitor Your Menstrual Cycle: Knowing your menstrual cycle and monitoring ovulation will help you pinpoint your fertile window for optimal intercourse timing.

12. Seek Medical Advice: If you have reproductive difficulties or have been trying to conceive for an extended time without success, check with a healthcare professional or a fertility expert for a full assessment and assistance.

13. Maintain open communication and emotional support with your spouse throughout your reproductive journey. Seek expert help if necessary.

14. Be Patient: Fertility may take time, so it's essential to be patient and avoid undue stress.

Consider Alternative treatments: Some people find complementary treatments such as acupuncture, herbal medicine, or chiropractic therapy beneficial in increasing fertility. Before attempting alternative remedies, consult with a healthcare practitioner.

7.5 Preparation for a Healthy Pregnancy

Preparing for a healthy pregnancy is making proactive efforts to improve your health and boost your chances of a healthy pregnancy. Here's a complete guide on good pregnancy planning:

1. Care Before Conception:

Consult a Healthcare Provider: Make an appointment with your healthcare provider or obstetrician to discuss your pregnancy plans. They may provide advice and handle any worries or medical issues.

Examine medicines: Talk to your doctor about your current medication, including over-the-counter and prescription prescriptions. During pregnancy, several drugs may need to be altered or changed.

Manage Chronic Concerns: Before conceiving, consult your healthcare practitioner to verify that any chronic health concerns, including diabetes, hypertension, or thyroid disorders, are well-managed.

Vaccinations: Check your immunization status since certain vaccines are necessary before pregnancy to protect you and your baby.

2. Food and nutrition:

Balanced Diet: Consume a diet rich in fruits and vegetables, whole grains, lean proteins, and dairy or dairy substitutes. As directed by your healthcare professional, take prenatal vitamins or folic acid supplements.

Folate: Folic acid is necessary for the prevention of neural tube malformations. Consume folate-rich meals and take a folic acid-containing prenatal vitamin.

Hydration: Drink plenty of Water and avoid coffee and sugary drinks.

3. Factors of Lifestyle:

Maintain a Healthy Weight: Achieve and maintain a healthy weight by exercising regularly and eating a well-balanced diet. Obesity and being underweight may both have an impact on fertility and pregnancy outcomes. Regular moderate-intensity exercise is recommended. Please consult your healthcare practitioner about your workout regimen to verify it is safe during pregnancy.

Avoid Harmful Substances: Stop Smoking, avoid drinking, and limit your exposure to pollutants and secondhand smoke.

Manage Stress: Engage in stress-reduction activities such as meditation, yoga, or deep breathing exercises.

4. Sexual and Reproductive Health:

When you're ready to conceive, stop using birth control techniques. After halting some treatments, your fertility may take some time to recover to normal.

Track Ovulation: Understand your menstrual cycle and ovulation to discover your viable window for improved intercourse timing.

5. Genetic Analysis:

Consider genetic testing to rule out any hereditary diseases or carrier status. Discuss the findings with a genetic counsellor to further understand the possible hazards.

6. Prenatal Care:

Begin prenatal treatment as soon as possible throughout your pregnancy. Regular check-ups with your healthcare practitioner are essential for monitoring your health and your child's growth.

7. Financial Preparation:

Check your insurance policy to see whether it covers maternity care. Begin saving for pregnancy-related costs.

8. Emotional Help:

If you are experiencing worry or stress due to pregnancy planning, seek emotional Help from friends, family, or support organizations.

9. Get Ready for Parenting:

Take parenting seminars, read books, and acquire pregnancy and parenting knowledge to feel better prepared for the adventure ahead.

10. Maintain Your Knowledge:

- Read trustworthy sources and talk with your healthcare practitioner to stay current on the newest prenatal care and pregnancy breakthroughs.

Appendices

Fertility Terminology Glossary

Understanding fertility-related terminology is critical when embarking on the route to parenting. Here's a list of often-used fertility terms:

Infertility is the failure to conceive after a year of regular, unprotected intercourse (or six months for women over 35) or the inability to terminate a pregnancy.

Fertility is defined as the inherent capacity to conceive and have offspring.

Ovulation is the monthly release of a mature egg from the ovaries in women of reproductive age.

Menstrual Cycle: The monthly hormonal cycle in women includes uterine lining shedding (menstruation) and egg release (ovulation).

Follicle: A fluid-filled sac inside the ovaries containing a developing egg.

Luteinizing Hormone (LH): A pituitary gland hormone that causes ovulation.

Progesterone is a hormone released by the ovaries during ovulation that helps to sustain the uterine lining and early pregnancy.

Estrogen is a hormone generated mainly by the ovaries that plays an essential function in the menstrual cycle and fertility.

Cervical mucus is a fluid released by the cervix that varies in consistency during the menstrual cycle and is essential for sperm movement.

BBT: The body's resting temperature, which increases slightly after ovulation, may be used to trace the menstrual cycle.

Follicle-stimulating hormone (FSH): A hormone that promotes follicle development in the ovaries.

IVF is a fertility technique in which eggs and sperm are mixed in a laboratory dish, and the resultant embryos are placed in the uterus.

Intrauterine Insemination (IUI): A reproductive technique that inserts washed and concentrated sperm directly into the uterus.

Ectopic Pregnancy: A pregnancy that develops outside the uterus, usually in the fallopian tube.

PCOS is a common hormonal condition in women characterized by irregular periods, ovarian cysts, and, in some cases, insulin resistance.

Endometriosis is a disorder in which tissue identical to the uterine lining develops outside the uterus, causing discomfort and infertility.

Miscarriage: The termination of a pregnancy before the 20th week of pregnancy.

Ovarian Reserve: The amount and quality of eggs a woman possesses as she ages.

Semen Analysis: A test determining the amount and quality of sperm in a man's sperm.

Fertility Preservation: Techniques such as egg freezing preserve fertility for future use.

Donor Egg: The use of another woman's eggs to treat infertility.

Surrogacy is the procedure through which a woman bears and delivers a baby on behalf of another person or couple.

Gestational Carrier: A woman who bears and delivers a kid but is not biologically related to the child.

Embryo Transfer: During fertility treatments, fertilized embryos are placed in the uterus.

Ovarian Stimulation: The use of drugs to stimulate the ovaries to generate many eggs.

Fertility Specialist: A doctor or reproductive endocrinologist specializing in fertility diagnosis and treatment.

Fertility Clinic: A medical facility that provides fertility-related diagnostic and treatment services.

Book Resources for Further Reading

- Toni Weschler's "Taking Charge of Your Fertility"
- Jean M. Twenge's "The Impatient Woman's Guide to Getting Pregnant"
- Jorge E. Chavarro, Walter C. Willett, and Patrick J. Skerrett's "The Fertility Diet" Websites:
- The American Society for Reproductive Medicine (ASRM) provides information on fertility, reproductive health, and fertility treatment standards.

The American Pregnancy Association Provides a multitude of pregnancy, fertility, and reproductive health information.

Resolve: The National Infertility Association Offers infertility support, education, and advocacy to individuals and couples.

Apps for Fertility:

The clue is a period-tracking app that includes fertility and ovulation information.

Flo: Monitors periods and ovulation and provides fertility insights and counselling.

Ovia Fertility: Offers individualized fertility forecasts as well as fertility monitoring tools.

Community Websites:

BabyCenter Community: An online community for women to discuss their fertility and pregnancy journeys. What You Can Expect Forums: Provides a space for women to interact and discuss fertility and pregnancy issues.

Podcasts:

The Fertility Friday Podcast: Discusses a variety of fertility, menstrual health, and natural contraception issues.

Beat Infertility Podcast: This podcast features genuine tales from individuals who have struggled with infertility and professional guidance.

Journals of Medicine:

Medical publications and databases such as PubMed provide access to academic research and fertility and reproductive health studies.

Support Groups in Your Community:

See if there are any local fertility support groups in your region. Individuals and couples may share their stories and seek assistance during in-person gatherings in many places.

Specialists in Fertility:

Consult a reproductive endocrinologist or a fertility expert for individualized advice and resources tailored to your unique circumstances.

Services for Genetic Counseling:

If genetic testing or counselling is advised, choose reputed genetic counselling institutes or healthcare practitioners.

Practitioners of Alternative Medicine:

Consider talking with complementary and alternative medicine practitioners specializing in fertility assistance, such as acupuncturists or naturopathic physicians.

Recipe Index Breakfast Recipes:

- Smoothie with Berries and Spinach
- Granola Oatmeal with Sliced Bananas and Walnuts and Greek Yogurt Parfait with Berries
- Eggs Scrambled with Spinach and Tomatoes
- Pancakes with Whole Grain Flour and Fresh Berries
- Oatmeal with Pumpkin Spice and Pecans
- Spinach, banana, chia seeds, and almond milk smoothie
- Pineapple and flaxseed cottage cheese

Lunch Ideas:

- Salad with Spinach and Lentils with Lemon-Tahini Dressing
- Lentil and Vegetable Soup with a Side Salad Chickpea and Vegetable Stir-Fry with Brown Rice
- Salad of Tuna with Mixed Greens and Olive Oil Caprese Salad with Vinaigrette, Fresh Tomatoes, Mozzarella, and Basil
- Soup with Butternut Squash
- Salad of Mixed Greens with Apples, Cranberries, and Walnuts
- Soup with Vegetables and Lentils

Dinner Ideas:

- Salmon Baked with Asparagus and Quinoa
- Grilled Lemon and Herb Chicken Breast

- Grilled Shrimp Skewers with Zucchini and Summer Squash
- Quinoa with black beans and Bell Peppers Stuffed
- Stir-fried tofu with Broccoli and Brown Rice Baked Cod with Roasted Brussels Sprouts and Quinoa
- Chicken Roasted with Root Vegetables (Carrots, Potatoes, and Parsnips)
- Beef Stew with Carrots and Potatoes Cooked Slowly

Recipes for Snacks:

- Hummus with carrot and cucumber sticks
- A handful of mixed nuts and a little apple
- Pear Slices with Almond Butter
- Bites of Watermelon and Feta Cheese
- Peaches with Cinnamon Sprinkled Celery Sticks with Peanut Butter Sliced Pear with Almond Butter Dark Chocolate and a Handful of Mixed Nuts

Recipes for Side Dishes:

- Side Dish with Quinoa
- Sweet potatoes with green beans, roasted
- Chili-Lime Butter Garlic Corn on the Cob Potatoes Mashed
- Acorn Squash Stuffed with Quinoa, Brussels Sprouts Sautéed with Bacon and Shallots
- Bruschetta with tomato and basil

- Maple Glazed Roasted Winter Squash

Dear Valued Customer,

I hope you are enjoying your newly purchased book! I am pleased that you decided to invest in my product and I thank you for that.

I understand that your time is valuable, and am grateful for any additional time you may be able to take to provide an honest review. I believe that customer feedback is invaluable and your opinions will help me create an even better product in the future.

I would be deeply appreciative if you could take a few minutes to leave an honest review under this book. I truly value your feedback and thoughts and would be honored to receive your insights on the way I can improve.

I appreciate your commitment to my product and thank you for taking the time to provide an honest review.

Best Regard

Dr. Katrina T. Doles

9 798861 305822